PREPARING FOR THE MRCP PART 2

CARDIOLOGY

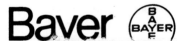
Robin M. Egdell

MA, MB, BChir, MRCP

Registrar in Cardiology
The Hillingdon Hospital
Uxbridge
Middlesex

with a foreword by
Prof. R. W. S. Campbell

Presented as a service to medical education by

Bayer

KLUWER
BOSTO

I extend my gratitude to Alison Rochelle, Molly Teoh, Yvonne Holloway and their respective departments for their invaluable assistance in the collation of the photographic material. Thanks are also due to my wife, Katie, for her many painstaking hours translating this work from illegible handwriting into megabytes.

Distributors

for the United States and Canada: Kluwer Academic Publishers, PO Box 358, Accord Station, Hingham, MA 02018-0358, USA
for all other countries: Kluwer Academic Publishers Group, Distribution Center, PO Box 322, 3300 AH Dordrecht, The Netherlands

A catalogue record for this book is available from the British Library

ISBN 0-7923-8869-0

Copyright

Published in the United Kingdom by Kluwer Academic Publishers,
PO Box 55, Lancaster, UK

Kluwer Academic Publishers BV incorporates the publishing programmes of
D. Reidel, Martinus Nijhoff, Dr W. Junk and MTP Press

Origination by Pindar, 1 Garstang Road, Preston, Lancashire, UK

Printed and bound in Great Britain by Pindar, 1 Garstang Road, Preston, Lancashire, UK

Foreword

This book is about passing an examination. There is no shame in that: Membership of the Royal College of Physicians is an essential passport to a hospital-based medical career. The MRCP examination comprehensively tests factual recall, intellectual agility and clinical acumen and it is a topical and ever-changing examination.

This book meets all of these challenges. Cardiological problems comprise a significant part of the practice of medicine and it is very appropriate that Robin Egdell has developed a specialist series of questions devoted to cardiology. In 41 superb questions with extended answers he covers the common and the uncommon, but throughout he maintains a sense of what is important. The book contains fine illustrations, be they electrocardiograms, X-rays, echoes, clinical photographs or nuclear magnetic resonance images. These illustrations and their associated questions embody the very essence of everyday cardiology. This book may have started out focused on a postgraduate examination. It goes further, but it covers the examination need with honours. As revision, as a self-test or as a reminder about the complexity and breadth of cardiovascular medicine, the questions offer much to those who may be long past their own personal encounter with MRCP. They are an extension of clinical practice. Whether it be the patient descriptions or the knowledge that the traces and images have come from patients, the challenges posed are neither artificial nor contrived; they are real life. This book is like an exciting outpatient clinic or ward round. It is challenging and rewarding. It is subliminal teaching; the kind that is painless and fun. Little wonder then that it is a superb preparation for the cardiological elements of MRCP Part 2.

Professor R. W. S. Campbell
Head, Department of Academic Cardiology
University of Newcastle
Freeman Hospital
Newcastle upon Tyne

Introduction

In addition to the accumulation of a vast quantity of knowledge, the MRCP exam demands the mastery of several different examination formats, from the multiple choice questions of the Part 1 to the viva exam that forms the final hurdle in the Part 2. The format which lends itself best to a book of this sort is that found in the written section of the Part 2 examination. Like those in the examination, the questions presented here may be divided into photographic material, data interpretation and case histories, though the boundaries between these subdivisions may sometimes blur and, for the sake of variety, the questions are not grouped according to type. Despite these similarities to the written section of the Part 2, the information contained in this book is applicable to all sections of the MRCP and should also be of value for the on-going post-graduate education of all physicians.

Those preparing for either part of the MRCP examination should not become discouraged upon finding some of the questions unexpectedly difficult. The standard is deliberately set somewhat higher than the exam. The intention is to educate, not to instil self-confidence and complacency. The reader who can answer all the questions correctly has learned nothing.

Robin M. Egdell

Glossary of Abbreviations

ACE - angiotensin converting enzyme

AF - atrial fibrillation

ALP - alkaline phosphatase

ALT - alanine transferase

ASD - atrial septal defect

AV - atrio-ventricular

Bili - bilirubin

Cr - creatinine

CT - computed tomography

CXR - chest X-ray

ECG - electrocardiogram

ESR - erythrocyte sedimentation rate

Gluc - glucose

GP - general practitioner

Hb - haemoglobin

HIV - human immunodeficiency virus

INR - international normalised ratio

IVC - inferior vena cava

IVS - inter-ventricular septum

K - potassium

LA - left atrium

LDL - low density lipoprotein

LV - left ventricle/ventricular

LVEDP - left ventricular end diastolic pressure

MCV - mean corpuscular volume

MRI - magnetic resonance imaging

MUGA - multiple uptake gated acquisition

MV - mitral valve

Na - sodium

PA - pulmonary artery

PCWP - pulmonary capillary wedge pressure

Plt - platelet count

PV - plasma viscosity

PW - posterior wall

RA - right atrium

RV - right ventricle

SA - sino-atrial

SHO - senior house officer

SLE - systemic lupus erythematosus

TFTs - thyroid function tests

U - urea

VF - ventricular fibrillation

VLDL - very low density lipoprotein

VSD - ventricular septal defect

WCC - white cell count

Q1.

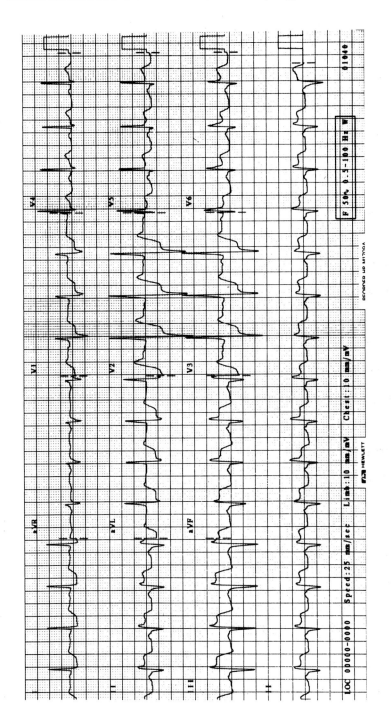

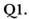

Q : What is the complete electrocardiographic diagnosis ?

A1.

A :   Acute inferior myocardial infarction with lateral and posterior extension

Acute inferior infarction should be an instant spot-diagnosis for the MRCP candidate. The relevant abnormalities are Q waves and ST elevation in the inferior leads, II, III and aVF. Closer inspection however will reveal the same changes present in the lateral leads, V5 and V6, though not in the "high lateral" leads, I and aVL, in this example. This indicates involvement of the lateral wall of the left ventricle.

More subtle still are the changes of posterior wall infarction. These consist of tall R waves, profound ST depression and (not in this example) tall peaked T waves in the early precordial leads V1-V3. Holding the ECG upside down and viewing it in a mirror will reveal the classic infarction pattern. The key element to this part of the diagnosis is the presence of tall R waves in these leads. These would not be features simply of anteroseptal reciprocal changes.

These ECG changes could result from occlusion either of a dominant circumflex artery or a dominant right coronary artery.

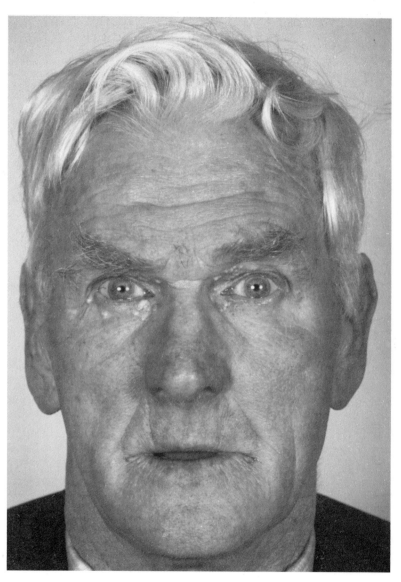

This gentleman has coronary artery disease, carotid artery disease, and peripheral vascular disease.

Q :   a) What physical sign is present ?
b) What is the likeliest biochemical diagnosis ?

A2.

A :   a) Xanthelasmata

   b) Type IIb hyperlipidaemia (Frederickson classification)

Although xanthelasmata can feature in a number of the hyperlipidaemias, they are most typical of mixed hyperlipidaemia (type IIb in the Frederickson classification). Other physical signs of the lipid disorders include a corneal arcus, tendon and tuberous xanthomata (IIa), eruptive xanthomata (I,IV,V), palmar crease xanthomata (III) and lipaemia retinalis (I,IV,V).

Type IIb hyperlipidaemia is characterised by raised cholesterol and triglyceride concentrations. Both LDL and VLDL levels are increased. The inheritance of the condition is complex, unlike the autosomal dominant familial hypercholesterolaemia (IIa). Some families appear to demonstrate an autosomal dominant inheritance, though with variable penetrance. In other families one can discern linkage with other hyperlipidaemias such as type IV.

Secondary hyperlipidaemias may form a type IIb pattern, diabetes being the commonest cause of this. Other causes of secondary hyperlipidaemias include obesity, alcoholism, nephrotic syndrome, renal failure, biliary disease and hypothyroidism.

Type IIb hyperlipidaemia, along with types IIa, III and IV, is an independent risk factor for atherosclerotic disease and therefore occupies a significant place in cardiological science.

Q3.

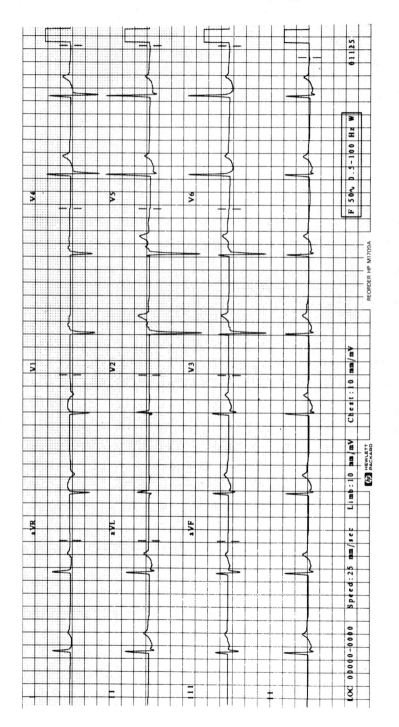

Q: What abnormality is evident?

A3.

A : Junctional rhythm

The baseline between adjacent ventricular complexes is entirely flat. The QRS complexes are narrow (less than 0.12 seconds) indicating that they originate from the bundle of His or above. Careful inspection of a number of leads, most clearly V2, reveals the atrial activity in this tracing. Some 60 milliseconds after the end of the QRS complex is a small deflection of about 40 milliseconds duration which is almost certainly a P wave. The same deflection can be appreciated in the inferior leads, II, III and aVF. In these leads, however, the deflection is negative (downwards). Normal atrial activation leads to positive P waves in the inferior leads, since the wave of depolarisation should travel inferiorly from the sinoatrial node to the atrioventricular node. In this example, atrial activation is therefore late and retrograde. Ventricular activation is normal but precedes atrial activation. These are the hallmarks of a junctional or nodal rhythm. The rate, a shade under 50 beats per minute, is typical of the AV node's intrinsic pacemaker activity. Although one may see junctional rhythm in normal subjects, particularly the young with high vagal tone, it may also be seen in the context of inferior ischaemia or infarction, or metabolic upset.

The lateral ST sagging in this example is non-specific and probably reflects the profound metabolic abnormalities which underlay the rhythm disturbance in this case.

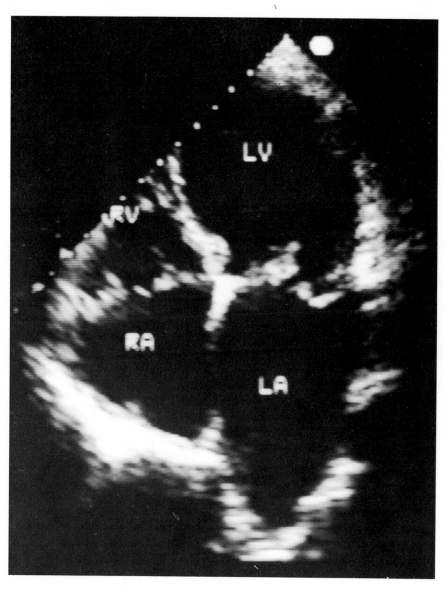

This fit young woman has a late systolic murmur.

Q :   What does her echocardiogram show ?

A4.

A : Mitral valve prolapse

This is an apical four-chamber echo view. The frame is taken during systole, as evidenced by the closed atrioventricular valves. Close inspection of the mitral valve reveals that one leaflet (the posterior) has prolapsed back behind the plane of the anterior leaflet. There is consequently a gap between the two leaflets and one does not need colour-flow Doppler to predict significant mitral regurgitation, accounting for the degree of left atrial enlargement.

Mitral valve prolapse (or "floppy mitral valve syndrome") is a common condition affecting up to 10% of the population. Usually it is an incidental finding on echocardiography, and is defined as systolic prolapse of one or both mitral leaflets behind the plane of the valve. Most cases will not be accompanied by regurgitation.

Mitral valve prolapse is said typically to affect tall, thin young adults, with a higher incidence in females. It is often accompanied by atypical chest pains or palpitations in the absence of documented rhythm disturbance. Mitral valve prolapse is said to occur in 50% of people with pathological anxiety and panic attacks, and the disorder can therefore present with a plethora of ill-defined symptoms. However, a proportion of patients with mitral valve prolapse do have demonstrable rhythm

√ **Q5.**

A 22–year–old man with a history of eczema was brought to the Accident and Emergency department after collapsing on the football field. According to witnesses, he remained unconscious for about five minutes, during which time some fitting activity was noticed. Upon regaining consciousness he denied chest pain or dyspnoea. His family history was incomplete, his father having died suddenly eighteen years earlier. However there was no history of ischaemic heart disease on his mother's side of the family.

The Casualty Officer thought she could hear two distinct systolic murmurs, but noted no other abnormal physical signs. His electrocardiogram showed sinus rhythm, P mitrale, a mean QRS axis of -47^0 and left ventricular hypertrophy with marked repolarisation abnormalities. Apart from a white cell count of 12.4×10^9/L, all routine blood tests were normal. The Casualty Officer arranged an urgent echocardiogram.

Q : a) ~ What did the echocardiogram show ?

b) What is the diagnosis ?

c) What other signs might have been elicited by more careful physical examination ?

d) What was the likeliest mechanism of the syncopal event ?

A5.

A : a)   Small left ventricular cavity

          Asymmetric septal hypertrophy

          Subaortic left ventricular outflow tract obstruction

          Systolic anterior motion of the mitral valve leaflets

          Mitral regurgitation

          Reduced diastolic compliance

     b)   Hypertrophic (obstructive) cardiomyopathy

     c)   Bisferiens pulse

          Double apical impulse

          Apical heave

          Fourth heart sound

          Accentuation of the murmur by manoeuvres that reduce peripheral resistance, e.g. rising from a squatting position

     d)   Ventricular tachycardia   *exercise*

Hypertrophic cardiomyopathy (it need not have a significant "obstructive" component) is inherited in an autosomal dominant pattern. Histologically, myocyte architecture is grossly abnormal, being arranged in whorls rather than sheets. Although the typical murmur is an ejection systolic murmur of left ventricular outflow tract obstruction, mitral regurgitation is a common accompaniment. Systolic anterior motion of the mitral valve leaflets is a characteristic finding best seen on M-mode echocardiography, and may result from the Venturi effect of the high velocity jet in the left ventricular outflow tract anterior to the mitral valve. It is probably this same phenomenon, interfering with normal coaptation of the mitral valve leaflets, which underlies the mitral regurgitation commonly seen.

Abnormal left ventricular relaxation leads to high left atrial pressures and a high incidence of atrial arrythmias. However, ventricular tachycardia is the more feared rhythm disturbance, and sudden death is not uncommon.

Q6.

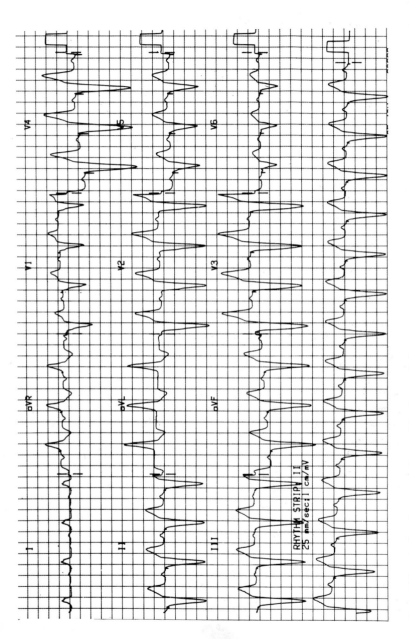

Q : What is the electrocardiographic diagnosis ?

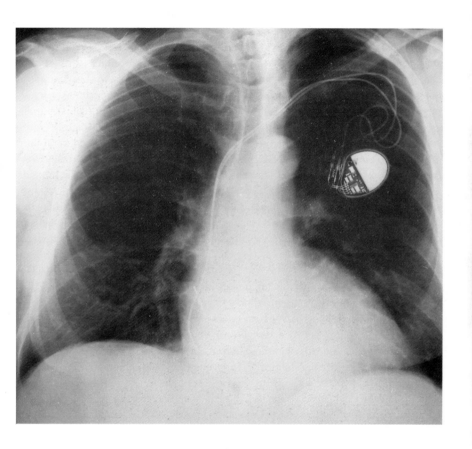

Some more data for the undecided...

A6.

A : Dual chamber pacemaker

The QRS complexes in the ECG are preceded by a sharp deflection of brief duration, best appreciated in lead V4. This is a pacing spike, generated by a permanent pacemaker. Because ventricular depolarisation originates from the apex of the right ventricle, the QRS complexes are broad and their mean axis is deviated to the left.

Despite the clear presence of a ventricular pacemaker, careful observation reveals atrio-ventricular concordance. Each pacing spike follows a normal P wave. This is characteristic of a dual chamber pacemaker. The atrial activity in this example is normal, generated by depolarisation of the sino-atrial node. The pacemaker senses this and stimulates ventricular contraction after an appropriate interval (160 milliseconds in this example). Both atrial and ventricular leads are capable of sensing and pacing. Thus if the spontaneous atrial rate falls below a pre-defined minimum, the pacemaker will pace the atria. Similarly, if AV conduction should occur normally, the ventricular activity will be sensed and the ventricular stimulus inhibited.

The X-ray confirms the ECG diagnosis. The pacemaker sits in a subcutaneous pocket below the left clavicle. Two leads run from this into the heart. One ends in the right ventricular apex. The other curls back on itself to lie anteriorly in the right atrial appendage.

Advantages of dual chamber pacing modes include the response of the ventricular rate to autonomic and adrenergic stimuli, via the SA nodal rate. Thus exercise will cause an appropriate increase in the ventricular rate. In addition, the normal temporal relationship between atrial and ventricular contraction may endow significant benefits in terms of cardiac output. In individuals with heart failure, the optimisation of ventricular filling by experimenting with different AV delays is possible.

Disadvantages of this pacing mode include increased cost and a more complex insertion procedure and follow–up. Later complications may arise, such as the theoretical risk of atrial tachyarrythmias being transmitted to the ventricles, or retrograde AV conduction resulting in a circus-movement tachycardia.

The following catheter data were obtained during invasive investigation of a 5–year–old boy with a harsh systolic murmur :

	Pressure (mmHg)	Oxygen saturation (%)
IVC	6	63
RA	7	65
RV	28/−1	84
PA	26/16	86
LV	104/6	100
Aorta	109/63	99

Q :   What is the diagnosis ?

A7.

A : Ventricular septal defect

The pressures recorded are normal. However there is a "step up" in oxygen saturation on the right side of the heart. This implies shunting of saturated blood from the left at ventricular level, i.e. a ventricular septal defect.

In this case the normal right-sided pressures indicate that the shunt has not had any detrimental haemodynamic effects. Often the loudest murmurs are produced by the smallest ventricular septal defects ("Maladie de Roger").

Congenital ventricular septal defects tend to occur in the membranous part of the septum, immediately below the atrio-ventricular valves. This contrasts with ventricular septal defects acquired following infarction, which occur much deeper in the muscular part of the septum, usually apically or inferoposteriorly. Small congenital ventricular septal defects frequently close spontaneously. This is partly a result of relative diminution of the size of the defect compared to the growing heart, and partly an ill-understood remodelling of the septal leaflet of the tricuspid valve, "plugging" the hole.

Q8.

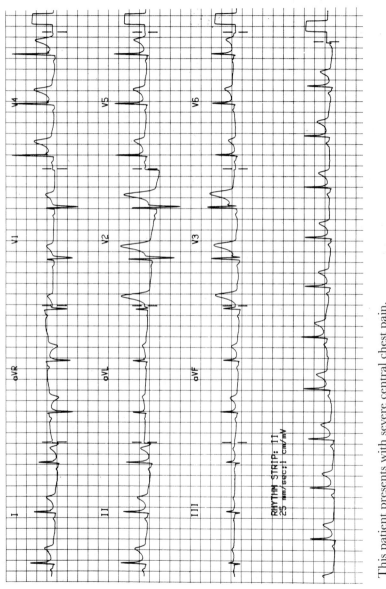

This patient presents with severe central chest pain.

Q: What is the diagnosis ?

A8.

A :   Pericarditis

There is widespread concave ST elevation. Although the appearances could be consistent with the very early stages of infarction in any one territory, the fact that several different territories are involved makes this highly unlikely.

The majority of acute pericarditis is viral in aetiology. The treatment of choice consists of bed rest and anti-inflammatory drugs. However, some would advocate close medical supervision in hospital since a small proportion of patients develop a significant pericardial effusion with the potential risk of tamponade. In practice this is rare.

A few patients go on to suffer recurrent episodes of pericarditis. This is probably an abnormal immunological response akin to Dressler's syndrome.

Other causes of pericarditis include acute pyogenic bacterial infections, tuberculosis, connective tissue disorders such as SLE and rheumatoid arthritis, acute rheumatic fever and uraemia.

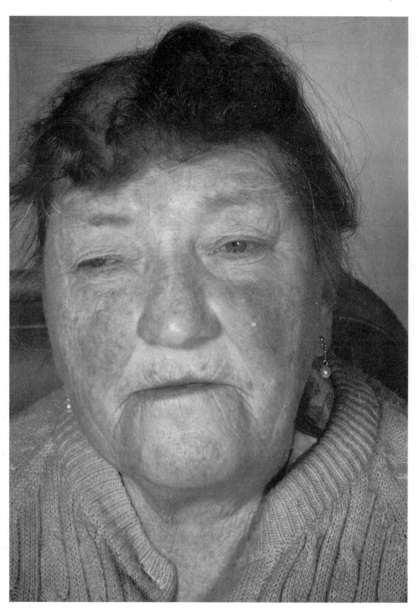

This woman presents with worsening exertional angina.

Q : What is the diagnosis ?

A9.

A :   Hypothyroidism

The coarse, "toad-like" facies, with periorbital myxoedema and thinning of the lateral portion of the eyebrows, is typical of hypothyroidism. Other clinical features include dry skin and hair, bradycardia, hypothermia and a goitre.

Hypothyroidism is a risk factor for coronary atherosclerosis, independent of the hyperlipidaemia which commonly co-exists. The management of angina in the context of hypothyroidism can be problematic. Thyroid replacement, by increasing heart rate and myocardial oxygen consumption, can worsen anginal symptoms, while the bradycardia and left ventricular systolic dysfunction which commonly accompany hypothyroidism may preclude the use of a number of anti-anginal drugs. These problems can usually be overcome by simultaneous introduction of L-thyroxine and a Beta-blocker, accompanied by very close monitoring of the patient's clinical state.

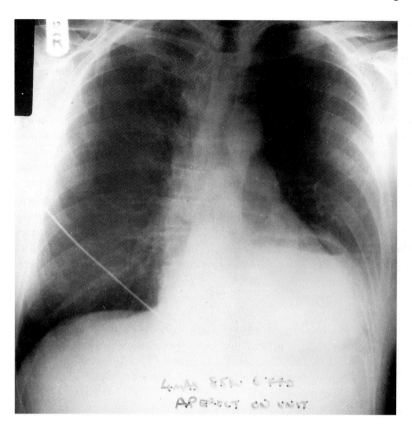

A 72–year–old man, with a long history of vague chest discomfort, is admitted with recent recurrent episodes of severe retrosternal pain at rest.

Q :   What does his chest X-ray show ?

A10.

A :   Hiatus hernia

Although the possibility of ischaemic heart disease cannot be excluded by chest radiography, this X-ray clearly shows a fluid level, with an associated gas bubble, behind the heart. These features are almost certainly within the stomach, herniated superiorly through the diaphragm.

This patient's subsequent endoscopy showed severe ulceration within the oesophagus and the herniated portion of the stomach.

Pain from the upper gastro-intestinal tract is one of the most frequently encountered mimics of ischaemic myocardial pain. The pain of oesophageal spasm in particular resembles angina, even to the point of radiation to the neck and arms. The pain of gastro-oesophageal reflux may be induced by exercise, because of an increase in intra-abdominal pressure. The development of pain when lying supine does not necessarily implicate reflux, since angina can also be brought on by adopting a horizontal posture ("decubitus angina").

The interaction between oesophageal pain and angina goes beyond simple mimicry. There is growing evidence of a link between oesophageal muscle tone and coronary arterial tone. It is clear that gastro-oesophageal reflux and oesophageal spasm can induce or exacerbate angina in patients with coronary artery disease. It is also possible that oesophageal spasm may trigger coronary artery spasm in individuals without coronary atheroma.

— **Q11.**

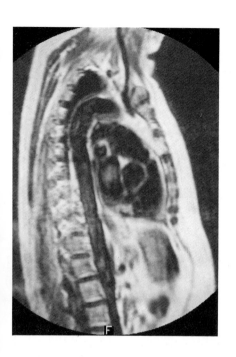

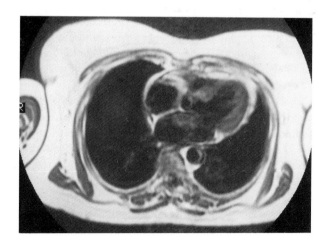

Q : a)   What is this investigation ?

b)   What does it show ?

A11.

A :   a)   Cardiac magnetic resonance imaging

         b)   Left atrial myxoma

Magnetic resonance imaging (MRI) is gaining favour as a very useful tool for depicting cardiac anatomy with high definition. Because of the ability of MRI to depict flow data, it has a place in the assessment of cardiac and vascular function as well as structure.

The two images here are longitudinal oblique and transverse images through the heart to show left atrium, mitral valve and left ventricle. They show a mass within the left atrial cavity, seen prolapsing into the left ventricle (these are late diastolic frames). This is most probably a myxoma.

Seventy-five percent of myxomas are found in the left atrium. The remainder are mostly right atrial. Occasionally a single myxoma is found in both atria, traversing a patent foramen ovale ("dumb-bell tumour").

The tumour is benign, consisting of small polygonal cells of uncertain origin, surrounded by a mucopolysaccharide-rich stroma. Although benign, the tumour is friable and pieces of it can readily embolise. Occasionally these emboli continue to grow ("macro-metastases").

The presentation of myxoma is most commonly with embolic phenomena. Alternative presentations include torrential mitral regurgitation from disruption of this valve, pulmonary hypertension from longstanding impairment of left ventricular filling, and a systemic illness with features of vasculitis and immune activation.

Cardiac auscultation in cases of left atrial myxoma commonly mimics mitral stenosis. The first heart sound is loud and may be double (not split – the second component is derived from the tumour itself, not tricuspid closure). There may be a low frequency mid-diastolic rumble. This may be preceded by a "tumour plop" in early diastole which mimics the opening snap of mitral stenosis, though is distinguished from it phonocardiographically by its later onset and lower frequency. It is also worth knowing that most patients with a myxoma will maintain sinus rhythm, whereas all but the young patients with significant mitral stenosis with be in atrial fibrillation.

√ **Q12.**

A girl of 11 was noted by the school doctor to have a cardiac murmur, but failed to attend the cardiology appointments arranged for her. She presented to her GP at the age of 27 following an episode of haemoptysis. Noticing the earlier events, the GP was relieved to discover her murmur had vanished. Shortly after being referred for respiratory assessment she came to cardiac catheterisation, with the following results :

	Pressure (mmHg)	Oxygen saturation (%)
IVC	19	52
RA	22	54
RV	120/14	55
PA	121/70	56
LV	112/11	77
Aorta	108/67	79

Q : What is the diagnosis ?

A12.

A : Eisenmenger's syndrome

The uncorrected left-to-right shunt, heard by the school doctor, has led to progressive pulmonary hypertension. The result of this is the development of systemic pressures within the right ventricle and subsequent reversal of the shunt. The right-to-left shunt remaining is evidenced by the desaturation of blood harvested from the left ventricle. One cannot determine from the data presented here whether the shunt is at atrial or ventricular level.

The symptoms of Eisenmenger's syndrome are those of right heart failure, arterial desaturation and polycythaemia. Haemoptysis is also a common accompaniment, possibly a result of small pulmonary infarcts.

The development of Eisenmenger's syndrome precludes surgical correction of the cardiac lesion. Closure of the shunt in the face of systemic pulmonary arterial pressures would lead to intractable right heart failure. Heart–lung transplantation offers some hope to these patients.

√ .**Q13.**

A 55–year–old male accountant with a history of hypertension and duodenal ulceration presents with tearing interscapular back pain and a new early diastolic murmur. A contrast-enhanced CT scan of his thorax confirms aortic dissection involving the ascending aorta and disrupting the aortic valve. Replacement of the aortic root with a Dacron graft and replacement of the valve with a Starr–Edwards prosthesis is successfully undertaken.

After an excellent initial convalescence, he returns for a follow–up appointment complaining of increasing lethargy, exertional dyspnoea and palpitations. His medication includes Warfarin, Methyldopa, Nifedipine and Ranitidine. Physical examination reveals a small haematoma related to his sternal scar, sinus tachycardia, an ejection systolic murmur and pale mucous membranes. No splenomegaly can be discerned.

Subsequent investigations yield the following results :

Hb–5.7 g/dL	Direct Coombs test negative	Serum iron decreased
MCV–69 fL	Faecal occult blood negative	Transferrin increased
WCC–12.1 x 10⁹/L	Urinary haemosiderin positive	Ferritin decreased
Plt–486 x 10⁹/L		
Blood film		ESR–27 mm
–Microspherocytes		INR–3.4
–Fragmented red cells		

Echocardiogram shows a well–functioning valve prosthesis

Q : a) What is the diagnosis ?

b) What is the treatment ?

A13.

A : a) Intravascular haemolysis

b) Iron replacement therapy

Repeat valve replacement

Fragmentation of erythrocytes on a prosthetic valve is an unusual complication of valve replacement, which does not necessarily imply haemodynamic dysfunction of the prosthesis. Although this usually manifests itself as a low-grade iron-deficiency anaemia, the phenomenon may occasionally cause clinically important anaemia.

The blood film may show erythrocyte fragments characteristic of intravascular haemolysis, while the iron studies will confirm the iron-deficient nature of the anaemia. Unlike extravascular haemolysis, during which iron is harvested and recycled, intravascular haemolysis is accompanied by renal loss of iron. This can be detected by microscopy of spun urine after appropriate staining – urinary haemo-siderosis.

Other possible explanations of this anaemia include gastro-intestinal blood loss secondary to peptic ulceration, exacerbated by anticoagulation, or alternatively auto-immune haemolysis related to Methyldopa. The negative faecal occult bloods and Coomb's test respectively suggest these are not the correct diagnoses.

Q14.

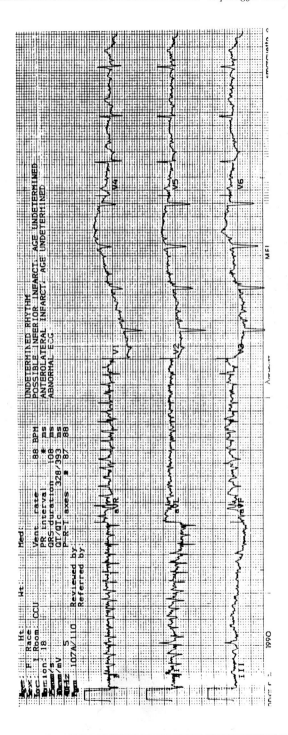

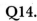

This woman was admitted directly from Casualty to the coronary care unit for DC cardioversion. The ECG computer does not know what to make of the cardiac rhythm.

Q: What is the diagnosis ?

A14.

A :   Normal sinus rhythm

Somatic muscle tremor

The electrocardiogram is designed simply to pick up changes in electrical potential between its electrodes. It possesses no device to isolate the heart's electrical activity specifically. Just as one commonly sees the ECG pick up the alternating current of a nearby infusion pump, one can also be fooled by electrical changes within the patient's skeletal muscle.

The rhythm in this example, when leads V1 to V6 are examined, is clearly a regular, narrow complex rhythm at a normal heart rate. It is probably sinus rhythm, though the muscle tremor in these leads obscures the atrial activity. The apparent complexes in the axial leads are very close together, having a rate in excess of 400 per minute. The complexes themselves are of odd and variable morphology. They are not of cardiac origin and are in fact derived from skeletal muscle activity. By counting squares backwards from the visible QRS complexes in V3, one can just identify the true cardiac activity in aVF.

This woman, who appeared extremely agitated and unable to speak, was admitted directly to CCU by the admitting medical team for urgent DC cardioversion. On reviewing her ECG, and after careful physical assessment, the on-call Cardiology team transferred her across to the psychiatric unit where she made a full recovery.

Q15.

A twenty–year–old medical student returns to England for the autumn term, after spending the summer working on his uncle's cattle farm in New Mexico. Five days after his return he presents to his GP with fever, severe frontal headache, mild photophobia and neck stiffness. He is promptly admitted to hospital, where examination of his cerebrospinal fluid reveals a moderate lymphocytosis. A diagnosis of viral meningitis is made and symptomatic therapy administered. He is discharged after six days, his symptoms much improved though with a persisting fever.

He returns to his GP three weeks later with unresolved malaise and a new symptom, namely a dry cough. His GP reassures him that this represents nothing more than a severe dose of 'flu, but organises a chest X-ray in any case. The X-ray is reported as showing scattered small areas of consolidation. Fearing a staphylococcal pneumonia, the GP once more arranges his admission to hospital, where he is treated with Amoxycillin, Flucloxacillin and Erythromycin. No organism is isolated from his blood cultures and his cough remains non-productive. While on the ward, he is noted to be mildly jaundiced. His liver function tests show hyperbilirubinaemia, moderately raised transaminases and a slightly high alkaline phosphatase. Serological tests for Hepatitis A, B and C and for Epstein-Barr virus and cytomegalovirus prove unhelpful. Hepatic ultrasound shows a slightly enlarged liver with a homogeneous texture. His ESR is 84 mm in the first hour. A percutaneous liver biopsy is taken and he is discharged home pending its results.

Ten days later his biopsy is reported as showing multiple granulomata. He is readmitted to hospital for further investigations, including a serum ACE level, a Mantoux test and HIV testing. On this occasion, the admitting house physician thinks she can hear a soft early diastolic murmur at his left sternal edge. Subsequent echocardiography shows a disrupted aortic valve with adherent vegetations, and mild aortic regurgitation. Blood cultures again prove sterile.

Q: a) What is the diagnosis?

b) What is the treatment?

A15.

A : a) Q Fever

b) Tetracycline derivatives

The triad of pneumonitis, endocarditis and granulomatous hepatitis is peculiar to Q fever, an uncommon infection caused by the micro-organism *Coxiella burnetii*. Though this microbe is tick-borne, it is usually acquired by humans directly from infected domestic farm animals. Q fever has been described in many parts of the world, though is most commonly seen in the southern United States.

Most infections are either subclinical or characterised by an acute febrile illness associated with severe headache. Occasionally the infection becomes chronic and may manifest itself as a pyrexia of unknown origin, chronic hepatitis or culture-negative subacute endocarditis. The aortic valve is that most commonly involved in the endocarditis and one occasionally sees an associated myocarditis.

Coxiella burnetii does not grow in conventional blood culture medium, but the diagnosis may be made by serology. Along with fungi, Rickettsiae, Brucella and mycobacteria, Coxiella should be specifically looked for in all cases of culture-negative endocarditis.

Like the closely related Rickettsiae, *Coxiella burnetii* is resistant to most of the commonly used antibiotics. It does however demonstrate sensitivity to the tetracyclines and protracted courses of these drugs are necessary to treat the chronic infection. Despite this the organism may sometimes prove remarkably resilient and viable organisms have been isolated from valve tissue months and even years after the initiation of treatment.

Q16.

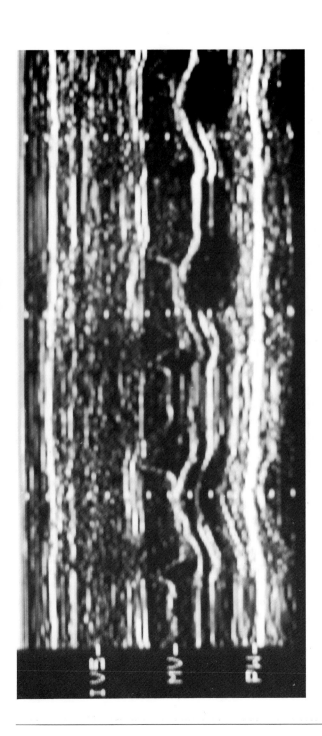

Q :

a) What is this investigation ?

b) What is the diagnosis ?

A16.

A : a)   M-Mode echocardiography

      b)   Hypertrophic cardiomyopathy

M-Mode echocardiography predates the two-dimensional echo but is still useful for depicting certain pathologies and certain aspects of cardiac function. The technique uses only a single beam of ultrasound, which is directed down through the area of interest. Solid structures reflect ultrasound and are seen as echogenic regions. Blood-filled cardiac chambers are seen as echo-free spaces. A single beam of ultrasound would produce only a vertical one-dimensional image, so the horizontal dimension of M-Mode is time. The pattern of the image therefore repeats itself over and over, each element of the pattern representing one cardiac cycle.

This is an example of M-Mode echocardiography through the mitral valve. This structure is seen opening in diastole, with an M-shaped configuration for the anterior leaflet, and a W-shaped configuration for the posterior leaflet. In systole the valve is closed, and the leaflets remain opposed and relatively motionless.

There are two abnormalities on this M-Mode which are characteristic of hypertrophic cardiomyopathy :

1)   Asymmetric septal hypertrophy (ASH). The interventricular septum (IVS) is grossly thickened. However, this is not simply left ventricular hypertrophy because the posterior wall (PW) of the left ventricle is of normal dimension (hence "asymmetric"). At the level of the mitral valve (MV), the interventricular septum lies immediately below the aortic valve. Hence marked septal hypertrophy here may lead to the subvalvar aortic stenosis of hypertrophic "obstructive" cardiomyopathy.

2)   Systolic anterior motion (SAM) of the mitral valve leaflets. As mentioned above, the diastolic excursion of the open mitral leaflets is normal. However, during systole, the leaflets should remain opposed and immobile, hence forming a straight line between adjacent M and W configurations. In this example, this line is not straight but bows anteriorly (towards the transducer). This abnormal motion of the closed mitral valve is possibly a result of the Venturi effect of a high speed jet of blood in the left ventricular outflow tract, anterior to the mitral valve leaflets. Whatever its cause, SAM, like ASH, is characteristic of hypertrophic cardiomyopathy.

Q17.

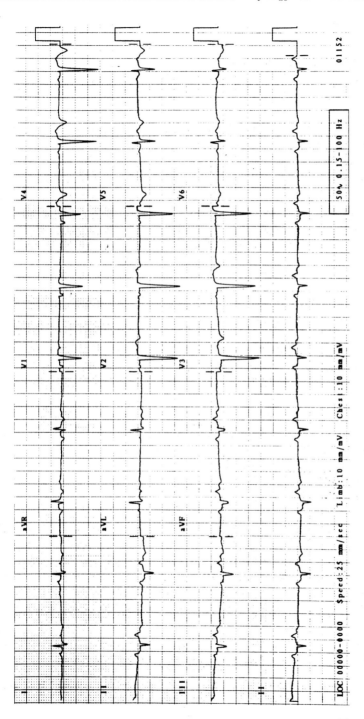

Q : This woman suffers from paroxysmal atrial fibrillation and atrial flutter.

What abnormalities are present on her ECG ?

A17.

A :   Non-conducted atrial bigeminy

Old anteroseptal and inferior infarction

Q waves in leads II, III, aVF, V1, V2 and V3 point to previous infarction in these territories. Persistent repolarisation abnormalities across the anterior leads may indicate this infarct to be relatively recent, though not necessarily.

More subtle is the disturbance of cardiac rhythm. At first sight it may appear to be a sinus bradycardia, with a rate of about 55 beats per minute. However, 0.32 seconds after the initiation of the normal P wave there is a second atrial deflection. This is best seen in the inferior leads and also therefore in the rhythm strip (lead II), where it is superimposed on the early part of the T wave.

Because this second atrial depolarisation is not equally spaced between adjacent sinus beats, it is an atrial extrasystole. Since every sinus beat is followed by such an extrasystole, it may be termed atrial bigeminy. The extrasystoles are not conducted presumably because the AV node remains refractory at this time.

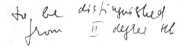
to be distinguished from II degree HL

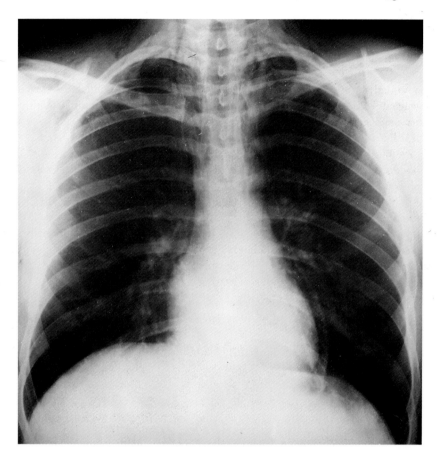

A 43–year–old man presents with central chest pain following a severe bout of gastro-enteritis. This is his chest radiograph.

Q : a) What is the diagnosis ?

b) What physical sign may be present on cardiac auscultation ?

A18.

A :   a)   Pneumomediastinum

       b)   Hamman's sign

The underlying pathology here is oesophageal rupture, secondary to severe, protracted vomiting. Air can be seen within the pericardial cavity, and extends up into the superior mediastinum. Because there is air on both sides of it, the parietal pericardium can be seen as a discrete line parallel to the heart border.

Air can also be seen delineating the soft tissues of the neck and axillae – surgical emphysema.

Hamman's sign is an audible "crunch" which occurs in time with the cardiac cycle and may alter with the patient's posture. Although it is said to occur occasionally in cases of small left-sided pneumothorax, the sign is virtually pathognomonic of pneumopericardium.

Q19.

A 34–year–old woman presents with a three month history of progressive lethargy, exertional dyspnoea and oedema. Her cardiac catheterisation yields the following data :

	Pressure (mmHg)	Oxygen saturation (%)
RA	a 16	68
	v 38	
RV	81/17	67
PA	78/52	63
LV	123/6	97
Aorta	127/71	96

Q : a) What is the diagnosis ?

b) What abnormal physical findings may be present ?

A19.

A :   a)   Primary pulmonary hypertension, tricuspid regurgitation

  b)   Raised venous pressure with prominent S (systolic) waves

   Parasternal heave

   Pulmonary component of S2 loud and delayed

   Pansystolic murmur at left sternal edge

   Oedema, hepatomegaly

Primary pulmonary hypertension is a condition which classically affects young and middle-aged women. It must be distinguished from pulmonary hypertension secondary to multiple pulmonary emboli.

The diagnosis may be suspected from the history, physical findings and typical X-ray appearances of large central pulmonary arteries with marked peripheral "pruning" of pulmonary vasculature. However cardiac catheterisation will usually confirm the diagnosis. The example here demonstrates high pressures throughout the right side of the heart, though pressures approaching systemic arterial pressure can be seen. Triscuspid regurgitation is the likely explanation of the high v wave pressure in the right atrium.

The physical signs are of pulmonary hypertension, right ventricular pressure over-load and right heart failure. Tricuspid regurgitation is a common accompaniment and, unlike that commonly seen in the normal low-pressure right heart, is frequently audible as a pansystolic murmur at the left sternal edge.

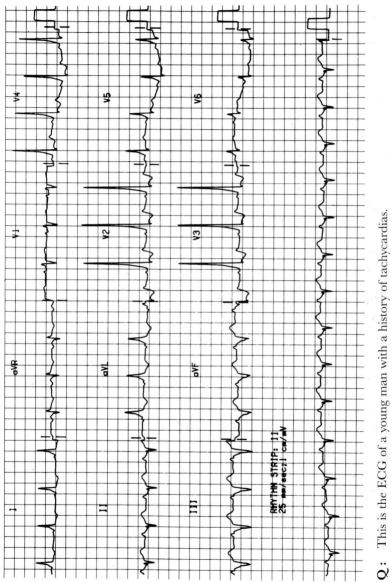

Q : This is the ECG of a young man with a history of tachycardias.

What is the diagnosis ?

A20.

A :   Type A Wolff–Parkinson–White syndrome

The PR interval is short, indicating rapid conduction from atria to ventricles. The first part of the QRS complex is slurred, leading to widening of the complex (ventricular pre-excitation). This initial slurring is referred to as the delta wave. These features, in the context of a history of tachycardias, are characteristic of Wolff–Parkinson–White syndrome (WPW).

Because the early precordial leads (particularly V2) are strongly positive, the initiation of ventricular activation must be coming from the left side of the heart (type A). In type B WPW, the accessory pathway lies in the right side of the heart and initial ventricular depolarisation is away from the right-sided leads.

The presence of ventricular pre-excitation renders interpretation of the remainder of the ECG impossible. In this example the left axis deviation, the tall R waves in V2 and V3 and the abnormal repolarisation (ST segments and T waves) across the anterior leads may all be part of the pre-excitation pattern. An ECG recorded after ablation of the accessory pathway might well prove entirely normal.

Wolff–Parkinson–White syndrome affects about 0.1% of the population. The pathology is an abnormal electrical connection between atria and ventricles, distant from the AV node. Multiple accessory pathways are not uncommon.

Although the most frequent presentation of WPW is with a re-entrant tachycardia, this rhythm can degenerate into AF. Because of the speed of conduction of the accessory pathway, the ventricular response rate in AF may be very fast (200–300 beats per minute) and may paradoxically be sped up by AV nodal blockers such as Digoxin or Verapamil. The danger of such rapid ventricular activity is the initiation of VF.

Electrocardiographically, the early part of the QRS complex is slurred and broad, the delta wave. This represents early depolarisation of myocardium distant from the rapidly-propagating specialised conducting system. The latter part of the QRS complex is narrow as the normal conduction, via the AV node and bundle branch system, "catches up". It is important to remember that ventricular pre-excitation will be apparent when the patient is in sinus rhythm or atrial fibrillation, but will not be seen when in a re-entrant tachycardia, as the anterograde conduction is only through the AV node in this situation.

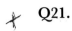

Q21.

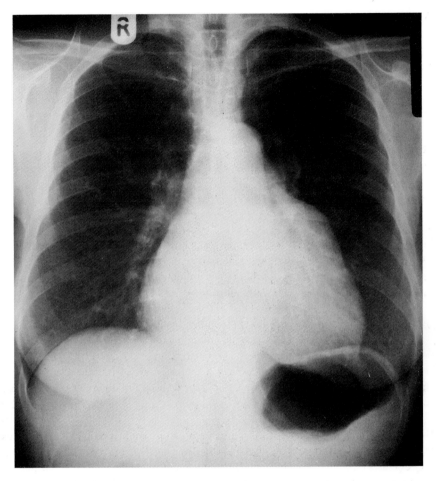

Q :   What does this X-ray show ?

A21.

A :   Left atrial enlargement

Left atrial enlargement may be inferred from a chest radiograph in three ways :

1)   Enlargement of the left atrial appendage. The bulge on the left heart border, inferior to the pulmonary arterial prominence, represents a large left atrial appendage.

2)   Double right heart border. A parallel shadow just medial to the right heart border can be seen, bestowing a "tram-line" appearance to this part of the cardiac outline. The second shadow represents the lateral border of the enlarged left atrium.

3)   Splayed carina. The bifurcation of the trachea into the right and left main bronchi lies immediately superior to the left atrium. Enlargement of this cardiac chamber therefore splays the bifurcation (the carina) more widely than normal. This is no more than a soft radiological sign, as there is no consensus on the normal limit of the bifurcation angle. Indeed some authorities dismiss its usefulness altogether. It should therefore only be used as corroborative evidence of left atrial enlargement.

Isolated left atrial enlargement is usually a consequence of mitral valve disease, particularly mitral stenosis. These X-ray appearances are therefore sometimes referred to as the "mitralised heart".

Radiologically, suspected left atrial enlargement can be confirmed by a lateral film during a barium swallow. The large left atrium can then be seen indenting the anterior aspect of the oesophagus. However, definitive confirmation of left atrial enlargement will be provided by echocardiography, which should also illuminate the underlying cause.

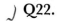

Q22.

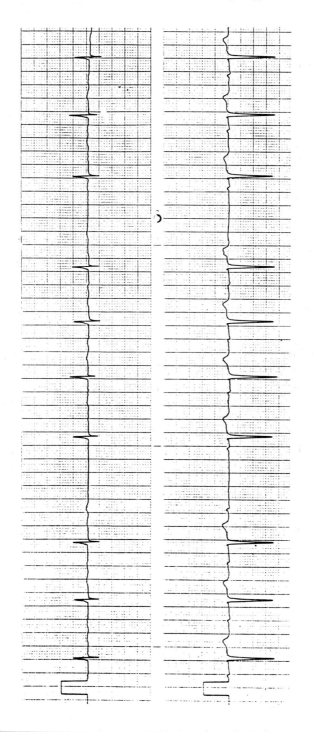

Q : What do these contemporaneous rhythm strips show ?

A22.

A : Type I 2nd degree heart block (Wenckebach)

The Wenckebach phenomenon can be recognised with ease from the lower of the two tracings. Here the PR intervals can clearly be seen to lengthen prior to the non-conduction of a P wave (visible after the T wave of complexes 3 and 10, but superimposed on the T wave of complex 7).

Although the upper tracing does not clearly show atrial activity, one can still infer Wenckebach block from it. This is because the RR intervals decrease fractionally prior to a missed complex, which is characteristic of the Wenckebach phenomenon.

That the pattern of "dropped" beats is not regular, as in this example, does not detract from a diagnosis of Wenckebach. A proportion of Wenckebach follows this shifting pattern. Longer rhythm strips may expose some predictability to this irregularity, and it is thought that such patterns are secondary to the interaction of different degrees of Wenckebach within different levels of the AV node.

The Wenckebach phenomenon is a common variant of normal, being present in 6% to 9% of "normal" 24 hour ECGs. It is particularly prevalent amongst the young, the athletic and those with high vagal tone. The block to conduction is usually within the AV node itself, rather than the His conduction system. As such it has an excellent prognosis, rarely causes symptoms and very infrequently requires permanent pacing.

Even when seen during inferior ischaemia or following inferior infarction, the Wenckebach phenomenon is usually transient and without haemodynamic consequence.

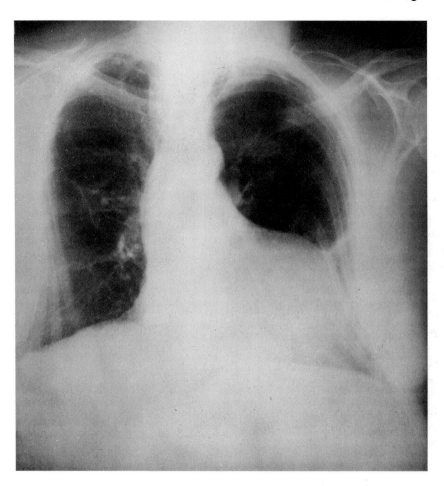

Question continued overleaf...

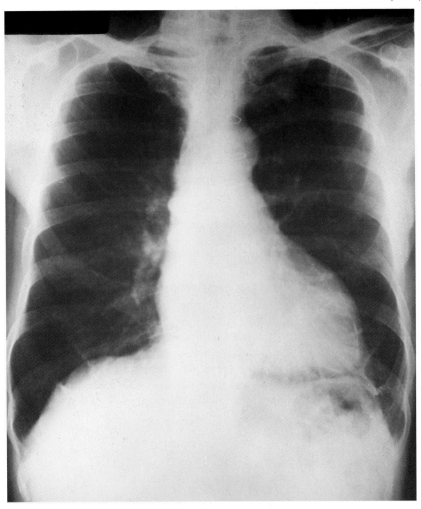

Q : The two patients whose X-rays are depicted here have the same cardiac diagnosis. What is it ?

A23.

A : Left ventricular aneurysm

In the first X-ray, the abnormal contour of the left heart border is suspicious of an LV aneurysm. The cup-shaped calcification seen in the second X-ray is hard to explain in any other way. When the two signs are seen in combination (i.e. a calcified bulge on the cardiac contour), the diagnosis is relatively secure. Confirmation can be sought with echocardiography, MUGA scanning, ventriculography or cardiac MRI.

LV aneurysms are said to complicate up to 15% of myocardial infarcts, though the exact figure depends on one's definition of an aneurysm. Structural aneurysms, rather than simple, dyskinetic "functional aneurysms", are probably much rarer than this. Their presence may be suspected by the persistence of ST elevation on the ECG, and the physical finding of a dyskinetic apical impulse.

LV aneurysms are most commonly anteroapical and are usually seen in the context of isolated occlusion of the left anterior descending artery (single vessel disease). Inferoposterior aneurysms are less common. Aneurysms probably take several months to develop following a myocardial infarction, as the ventricle "remodels".

Although 50% of LV aneurysms contain thrombus, embolism from this is unusual and oral anticoagulants will usually be sufficient to prevent clinical problems. More troublesome complications of a left ventricular aneurysm include left ventricular failure, poorly controlled angina and recurrent ventricular tachycardia. If any of these occur and prove resistant to medical therapy, surgical removal may be undertaken – an aneurysmectomy.

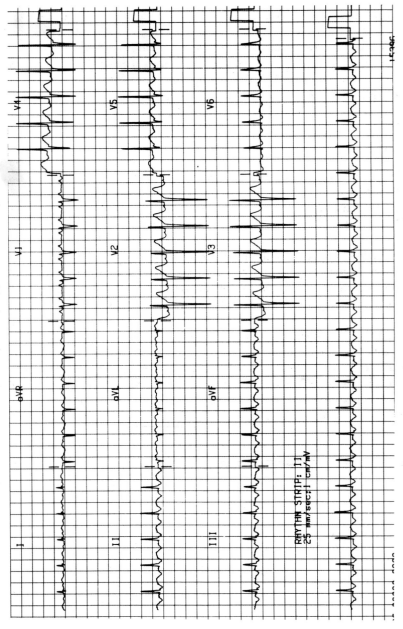

RHYTHM STRIP: II
25 mm/sec;1 cm/mV

Q: What is the electrocardiographic diagnosis ?

A24.

A :   Atrial flutter with 2:1 block

The classic saw-tooth waves of atrial flutter are only easily appreciated when the ventricular response rate is relatively slow. With 2:1 conduction, it may be difficult to pick out these flutter waves amongst the QRS complexes and T waves. However, in any regular, narrow complex tachycardia at or about 150 beats per minute, the possibility of atrial flutter must be considered.

The flutter waves in this example can be discerned on close inspection. In leads II, III and aVF the typical saw-tooth appearance is present. This may be appreciated better by looking at the ECG from either end with the paper angled downwards, thereby foreshortening the image. This technique renders the QRS complexes less obvious and enhances one's appreciation of the baseline.

Typical appearances of flutter are present in leads V1 and V2 also. In V1, what appears to be a normal P wave (if with a rather short PR interval) is mirrored by an identical deflection just after the QRS complex. In V2 this second atrial deflection is seen as a notch on the upstroke of the T wave. From this the atrial rate can be calculated to be around 300 beats per minute.

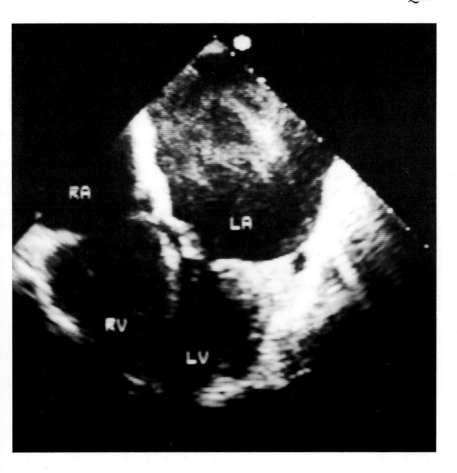

Q : a)   What precisely is this investigation ?

b)   What two abnormalities are present ?

c)   What is the diagnosis ?

A25.

A : a) Transoesophageal echocardiography

b) Spontaneous echo contrast in the left atrium

Thickened domed mitral valve with a restricted orifice

c) Mitral stenosis

A reasonable familiarity with standard echo views should alert one to the fact that this is not transthoracic echocardiography. Equally, the remarkably high image definition would be exceptional for a standard surface echo. This image is derived from a transoesophageal probe. On any echo, the transducer position is represented by the apex of the triangle that forms the whole image. Here the left atrium is at the apex, only a short distance from the transducer. The probe therefore lies within the oesophagus, immediately posterior to the heart.

This frame is taken during diastole, as evidenced by the open tricuspid valve. The mitral valve orifice however is very small and the valve itself is thickened and tethered. This is rheumatic mitral valve disease. The typical "domed" configuration of the rheumatic mitral valve during diastole is well shown here.

Spontaneous echo contrast ("smoke") is rarely seen on transthoracic echo, but commonly seen on transoesophageal. It represents stasis and sluggish flow of blood, and is probably caused by microaggregation of erythrocytes. In some situations, for example prior to DC cardioversion, the presence of left atrial smoke is thought to have the same implications as the detection of formed thrombus.

Mitral stenosis is almost always rheumatic in origin. It can be seen in the context of complex congenital heart disease but one is unlikely to encounter this in the MRCP clinical examination. The physical signs to elicit include a mitral facies (malar flush), atrial fibrillation, a tapping apex beat, a loud first heart sound, an early diastolic opening snap and a low frequency mid-diastolic murmur. Presystolic accentuation of the murmur is confined to those patients (usually the younger ones) who remain in sinus rhythm. If pulmonary hypertension has supervened, a right ventricular heave, a loud (and sometimes palpable) pulmonary second sound and the Graham Steele murmur of pulmonary regurgitation may be present. The severity of the stenosis can be assessed clinically by the delay between the second heart sound and the opening snap (inversely proportional to the left atrial pressure) and the duration of the murmur.

Q26.

A six–month–old girl with cyanosis is referred for cardiac catheterisation. The following figures are obtained :

	Pressure (mmHg)	Oxygen saturation (%)
IVC	10	49
RA	8	52
RV	96/6	56
PA	16/11	60
LV	94/7	92
Aorta	95/68	76

Q :   What is the diagnosis ?

A26.

A : Fallot's tetralogy

Fallot's tetralogy is the commonest cyanotic congenital heart lesion. The "tetralogy" consists of pulmonary stenosis (at infundibular, valvar or pulmonary arterial level), an unrestrictive VSD, a large aortic root which is shifted to the right and therefore overrides the VSD, and right ventricular hypertrophy. Embryologically, however, the "tetralogy" probably arises from a "monology" – the unequal division of the truncus arteriosus into right and left. This explains the failure of the truncal septum to meet the interventricular septum, and the size and position of the aortic root. Hypertrophy of the right ventricle is the predictable consequence of both pulmonary stenosis and free communication with the high-pressure left heart.

The data here illustrate the high right ventricular pressures and pulmonary stenosis (compare the systolic pressures in the right ventricle and pulmonary artery – these should be identical). The right-to-left shunt at high ventricular level is demon-strated by the desaturation of aortic blood as compared with blood harvested from the body of the left ventricle. As is often the case, there is some bi-directional flow across the shunt. There is also a step-up in right-sided saturations between right atrium and pulmonary artery, indicating some left-to-right shunting.

Clinical features in the neonate are usually confined to arterial desaturation (often with unnerving cyanotic spells) and the pulmonary stenotic murmur. Later in life, clubbing, the characteristic squatting posture, and problems associated with right-to-left shunting, such as polycythaemia and cerebral abscesses, may be seen. This latter picture is now unusual because of early diagnosis and successful surgical treatment.

Palliative surgery involves fashioning a left-to-right shunt above the level of the ventriculo-arterial valves. The Blalock–Taussig shunt consists of a subclavian artery anastomosed to the corresponding pulmonary artery. The Waterston shunt consists of an aorto-pulmonary window fashioned between the ascending aorta and the right pulmonary artery. The Potts shunt is a similar window between the descending aorta and the left pulmonary artery. These procedures will usually simply be holding measures prior to definitive surgical correction, during which the VSD is closed with a patch and the pulmonary stenosis relieved. The most favourable timing of corrective surgery is a matter of controversy.

Q27.

A 71–year–old woman, who has been on iron therapy for several years for recurrent anaemia, presents to Casualty following a collapse at home. She admits to a week's history of melaena but has not suffered any other abdominal symptoms. Her medications include ferrous sulphate and non-steroidal anti-inflammatory agents.

Physical examination reveals pallor, a blood pressure of 100/80 and a quiet systolic murmur. Careful abdominal examination is entirely normal. Rectal examination confirms the presence of melaena. Initial investigations show her haemoglobin concentration to be 6.7 g/dL with a microcytic blood film. Her electrocardiogram is abnormal, with tall R waves and T wave inversion in the lateral leads.

Subsequent endoscopy of the upper gastro-intestinal tract is surprisingly normal, and colonoscopy also fails to identify a source of bleeding. Echocardiography is undertaken to confirm the admitting SHO's impression that the systolic murmur is a flow murmur consequent upon anaemia. This investigation however reveals left ventricular hypertrophy and a maximum systolic transaortic pressure gradient of 90 mmHg. Realising the diagnosis, the SHO requests an investigation which does identify the source of bleeding.

Q : a)   What investigation does the SHO request ?

b)   What does it show ?

c)   What is the diagnosis ?

d)   What form of treatment would you advise in order to prevent further gastro-intestinal blood loss ?

A27.

A : a)   Mesenteric angiography

       b)   Abnormal vessels in the distribution of the superior mesenteric artery

       c)   Heyde's syndrome

       d)   Aortic valve replacement

Heyde's syndrome is the association of gastro-intestinal angiodysplasia, usually of the small bowel, with aortic stenosis. Although there is a school of thought that the "syndrome" is nothing but the chance association of two unlinked conditions, this case is far from proven. Particularly convincing evidence for the link comes in the form of numerous case reports of aortic valve replacement "curing" the gastro-intestinal blood loss.

The failure to diagnose the valve lesion in the case described here derives in part from a physical examination with too much gastro-intestinal emphasis, but also from the invalid conclusion that a quiet murmur precludes significant valvular disease. The murmur of aortic stenosis need not be loud, particularly when the stenosis is severe and when the left ventricle is failing. When considering the diagnosis of aortic stenosis, considerable emphasis should be placed on the "peripheral" physical signs, namely the pulse character, the pulse pressure, the systolic blood pressure, the nature of the apex beat, the presence or absence of a palpable thrill, and the volume and timing of the aortic component of the second heart sound.

Echocardiography allows assessment of transvalvar pressure gradients by the mathematical manipulation of peak flow velocities. When a valve is open, there should be no substantial pressure gradient across it. In the case of the aortic valve, this value should be less than 10 mmHg. Figures over 50 mmHg indicate severe stenosis. Although the example cited here fits into this category, it is not uncommon to see transaortic gradients well in excess of 100 mmHg.

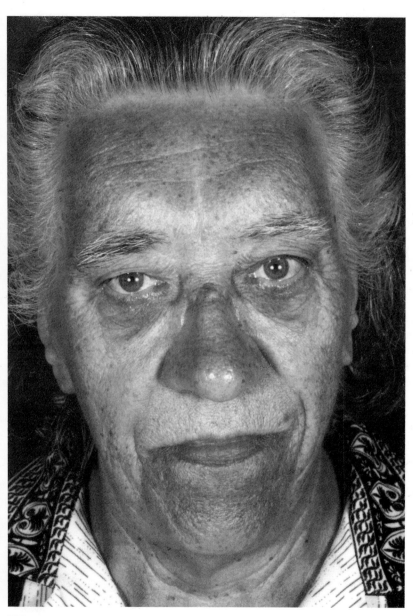

This woman presents in congestive cardiac failure.

Q :   What is the diagnosis ?

A28.

A : Acromegaly

Acromegaly, the result of excessive growth hormone secretion by a pituitary adenoma, is an uncommon cause of a dilated cardiomyopathy. The physical signs apparent in this case are prognathism, a prominent supraorbital ridge, coarse features and coarse, oily skin. An acromegalic facies however should be a pattern-recognition "spot diagnosis" for the serious MRCP candidate.

Other clinical features of acromegaly include macroglossia, spade-like hands, bilateral temporal hemianopia, diabetes, hypertension, pseudogout and features of hypopituitarism.

The diagnosis is made by growth hormone estimation during a glucose tolerance test, and by imaging the pituitary fossa by CT or MRI scanning.

Although bromocriptine and irradiation are conservative treatments sometimes used for palliation or adjunct therapy, surgical excision of the tumour forms the mainstay of management.

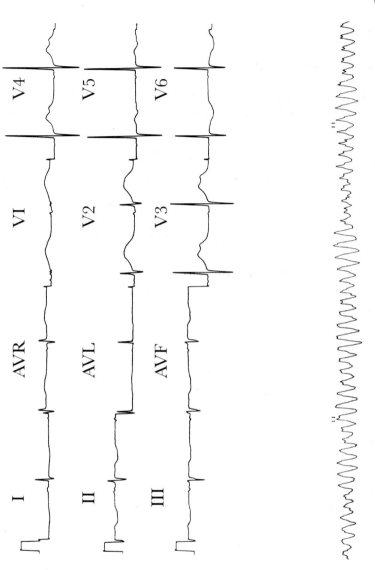

This 12-lead ECG and the accompanying rhythm strip were recorded from a gentleman whose only symptom was occasional syncopal events.

Q : What is the diagnosis ?

A29.

A :   Torsade de pointes

   Long QT interval

The 12-lead ECG, as well as showing marked sinus bradycardia, demonstrates a prolonged QT interval. The QT interval is the time from the beginning of ventricular depolarisation (the first deflection of the QRS complex) to the end of ventricular repolarisation (the end of the T wave or U wave if present). The QT interval shortens with increasing heart rate. Therefore, to determine whether a QT interval is normal or not, one needs to correct the value for heart rate (the QTc). QTc is calculated by dividing the measured QT interval (in seconds) by the square root of the RR interval (in seconds). The upper limit of normal for QTc is 0.44 seconds. The QTc in this example is substantially prolonged at 0.63 seconds (as measured in V3). Note also the prominent U waves in V3 and V4.

The rhythm strip shows a broad complex tachycardia. However, the morphology of the complexes is continually shifting such that the QRS axis appears to twist ("torsade") around the baseline. This is torsade de pointes ventricular tachycardia. It is almost exclusively seen in the context of a long QT interval. Probably it is the variability ("dispersion") of repolarisation times in different parts of the myocardium, rather than the duration per se, which predisposes to this tachycardia.

Common causes of long QT and torsade de pointes :

   Hypokalaemia
   Hypomagnesaemia
   Hypocalcaemia
   Hypothermia
   Bradycardia from any cause
   Antiarrhythmic drugs, particularly classes Ia and III
   Antipsychotic medication
   Congenital syndromes – Romano–Ward
                                     – Jervell–Lange–Nielsen

The arrhythmia is usually short-lived and self-limiting. However, sudden death can occur. In the emergency situation beta-blockers, magnesium, bretylium and over-drive pacing may be tried. Except in the case of the congenital long QT syndromes, the mainstay of treatment must consist of correction of the predisposing cause.

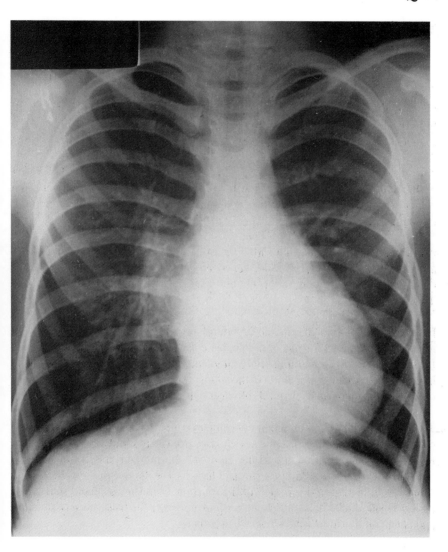

This boy has hypertension and a systolic murmur.

Q : a)   What does his chest radiograph show ?

      b)   What is the diagnosis ?

A30.

A : a) Rib notching

     b) Aortic coarctation

Although aortic coarctation often results in notching of most of the ribs, one can also see more localised patterns of notching. In this example, the inferior surfaces of both fifth ribs show notching, more marked on the left. Rib notching results from significant enlargement of intercostal arteries which act as collateral vessels.

The less common radiological sign of aortic coarctation is the "3 sign". This refers to the outline of the aorta immediately below the aortic knuckle, and represents the coarctation sandwiched between pre- and post-stenotic dilatations. (This sign is not evident in this example.)

Aortic coarctation is associated with a bicuspid aortic valve (in up to 80% of cases according to some studies), and hence co-existing calcific aortic stenosis or regurgitation. Coarctation is the commonest "cardiac" defect in patients with Turner's syndrome.

Physical signs are those of systemic hypertension in the upper part of the body, with additional radiofemoral delay and palpable collateral vessels around the scapulae. In the MRCP short case examination, radiofemoral delay must be sought routinely in the cardiovascular examination of the younger patient. Coarctation becomes very difficult to diagnose correctly if this physical sign is missed.

The murmurs of aortic coarctation are complex, since the bicuspid aortic valve, the coarctation itself and the collateral vessels may give rise to systolic murmurs. Aortic regurgitation may be present and the "systolic" murmurs arising from collaterals may be delayed and overlap into cardiac diastole. For the purposes of the MRCP clinical examination, a description of the murmur or murmurs should suffice and the candidate should be seen to listen for murmurs over the back, since coarctation and collateral murmurs will be heard better there.

Q31.

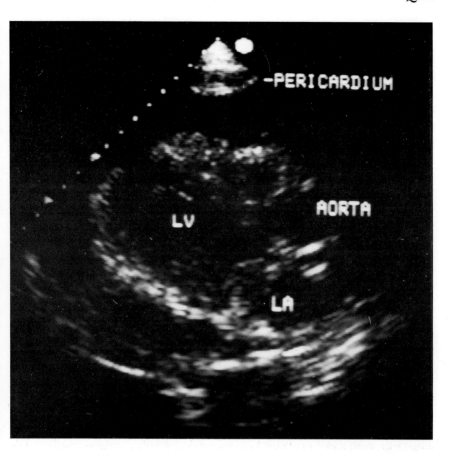

Q :   What is the abnormality ?

A31.

A :   Pericardial effusion

This is a parasternal long-axis echocardiographic view of the heart. The heart is surrounded by a large echo-free space. This is a pericardial effusion.

Causes of pericardial fluid include viral, bacterial or tuberculous pericarditis, uraemia, auto-immune disorders, trauma (including cardiac surgery), post-infarction, heart failure and malignancy. Haemopericardium is usually the result of rupture of part of the heart or aortic root and is seen post-infarction, after severe chest trauma and complicating aortic dissection.

The danger of an increasing pericardial effusion is cardiac tamponade. In slowly accumulating effusions, a large volume of fluid may be accommodated in the pericardium without embarrassing cardiac function. Rapidly accumulating pericardial fluid (for example the haemopericardium of post-infarct ventricular rupture) may lead swiftly to cardiac tamponade and electro-mechanical dissociation with as little as 100 millilitres of blood in the pericardium.

Symptoms of tamponade include dyspnoea, dizziness and collapse. Patients occasionally complain of a sensation of precordial pressure. The predominant physical signs of cardiac tamponade are those of shock, with pallor, cyanosis, sweating, tachycardia and hypotension. The quick-witted clinician will look for the more subtle signs suggestive of tamponade, such as pulsus paradoxus, a raised jugular venous pressure with a prominent X descent in the wave form and a positive Kussmaul's sign, an absent apex beat and quiet or inaudible heart sounds.

The chest radiograph may show an enlarged, "globular" cardiac shadow. The electrocardiogram may show small-voltage QRS complexes or electrical alternans. Echocardiography is usually diagnostic.

Emergency treatment of acute cardiac tamponade involves pericardial aspiration with a spinal needle and the largest syringe available. Given time, the more controlled and sterile positioning of a formal pericardial drain is preferable. Later management depends on the underlying cause, but may include the surgical fashioning of a pericardial window or pericardiectomy.

Q32.

The following catheter data are obtained from a 21–year–old woman with dyspnoea :

	Pressure (mmHg)	Oxygen saturation (%)
IVC	13	67
RA	14	80
RV	51/7	85
PA	53/31	84
PCWP (end diastolic)	17	
LV	134/3	99
LVEDP	6	
Aorta	135/86	99

Q : What is the diagnosis ?

A32.

A : Lutembacher's syndrome

The catheter data reveal two abnormalities. The step-up in saturation at atrial level implies an ASD. Additionally, however, there is a gradient between the end-diastolic PCWP and the LVEDP. This gradient, in practice demonstrated by simultaneous pressure tracings from a wedged pulmonary artery catheter and a left ventricular catheter, indicates mitral stenosis.

The combination of an ASD and mitral stenosis is referred to as Lutembacher's syndrome. Although both elements may be present at birth, the mitral stenosis frequently seems to be acquired later in life. The effect of developing mitral stenosis is an increase in left atrial pressure and consequently worsening of the left-to-right shunt.

It is not clear whether the two elements of Lutembacher's syndrome are always of the same aetiology, or whether occasionally acquired rheumatic mitral stenosis simply exposes a previously asymptomatic ASD.

Q33.

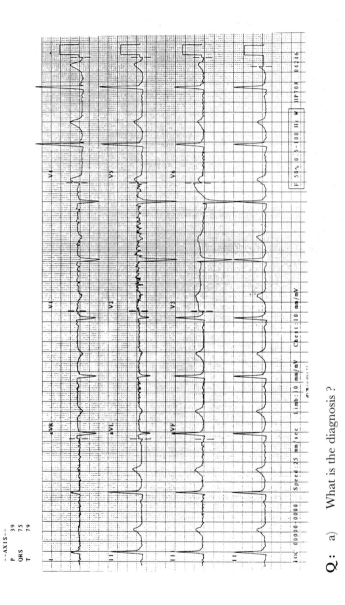

Rate 52
PR 184
QRSD 123
QT 601
QTc 559

--AXIS--
P 39
QRS 75
T 79

Q:

a) What is the diagnosis ?

b) What five ECG abnormalities support your diagnosis ?

A33.

A : a)   Hypothermia

        b)   Sinus bradycardia

              J waves

              Muscle tremor

              Widened QRS

              Long QTc

Sinus bradycardia is a frequent finding in significant hypothermia. One may also see delayed AV conduction (a prolonged PR interval). Atrial fibrillation may alternatively be present.

J waves are abnormal deflections at the end of the QRS complex (the J point – the junction between the QRS complex and the ST segment). They are characteristic of hypothermia, but need not be as obvious as in some textbook examples. Here they are best seen in lead V4, but inspection of almost all leads reveals abnormal slurring of the J point.

Skeletal muscle tremor causes artefactual irregularity of the baseline. Here this is best seen in lead V2. The maintenance of the shivering response is probably a favourable prognostic sign.

Hypothermia slows all bodily metabolic processes. Both cardiac depolarisation and repolarisation are similarly affected, resulting in wide QRS complexes and prolonged QTc (QT interval corrected for heart rate). These values are provided by the ECG computer in this example.

Q34.

A woman of 82 is admitted to the ward because of failure to cope at home. She has complained of worsening exertional dyspnoea for several weeks, but more recently has become mildly confused. Her previous history includes borderline hypertension, bilateral total hip replacements and an anterior resection of a Duke's B carcinoma ten years ago. She normally takes a thiazide diuretic and laxatives.

Physical examination reveals normal sinus rhythm, a blood pressure of 162/96, normal arterial and venous pulsations, a fourth heart sound but no cardiac murmurs. She has moderate peripheral oedema. She has a few fine crepitations at her lung bases. Abdominal examination reveals a palpable spleen tip and some inguinal lymphadenopathy. She has evidence of peripheral sensory loss in a "glove and stocking" distribution.

Investigations yield the following results :

Na – 136 mmol/L	Hb – 8.7 g/dL	Bili – 7 μmol/L	**Urine dipstick :**
K – 2.9 mmol/L	WCC – 8.9 x 10⁹/L	ALT – 22 IU/L	Blood +
U – 7.6 mmol/L	Plt – 94 x 10⁹/L	ALP – 143 IU/L	Protein +++
Cr – 97 μmol/L	PV – 2.3 mPa	Protein – 72 g/L	Glucose 0
Gluc – 8.4 mmol/L		Albumin – 24 g/L	
		TFTs – Normal	

CXR – Mild pulmonary congestion
     – Normal cardiac silhouette
ECG – Normal

Echocardiography shows a restrictive left ventricular inflow pattern and a small left ventricular cavity. There are bright acoustic reflections from the myocardium, especially in the interventricular septum, while the interatrial septum is markedly thickened.

Bone marrow examination reveals an excess of mature lymphocytes, plasma cells and immature lymphoid cells.

Q : a) What is the cardiac diagnosis ?

     b) What is the underlying diagnosis ?

A34.

A : a)   Cardiac amyloidosis

     b)   Systemic AL amyloidosis secondary to Waldenstrom's macroglobulinaemia

Infiltration of myocardium by amyloid protein leads to restrictive ventricular dysfunction. The abnormality of ventricular function is largely diastolic, early diastolic filling being rapid but truncated. This is best assessed echocardiographically by the Doppler pattern of mitral inflow and by ventricular wall motion on M-mode. The amyloid protein itself can be seen on the 2-D images as bright "speckling" within the myocardium, particularly in the septum.

Amyloidosis of the AL type classically causes macroglossia, cardiac failure, peripheral neuropathy and proteinuria. It may be primary, or secondary to abnormal immune protein production in conditions such as myeloma or Waldenstrom's macroglobulinaemia. Congo red is the stain used to demonstrate amyloid deposits in biopsies of tissues thought to be affected, or in the more easily obtainable rectal biopsy.

Waldenstrom's macroglobulinaemia is caused by clonal production of IgM by a functioning B-cell lymphoma. Apart from the clinical features of the lymphoma itself, the excess of plasma IgM can lead to hyperviscosity. This may present as confusion, neurological dysfunction or heart failure, and results in a high ESR and plasma viscosity.

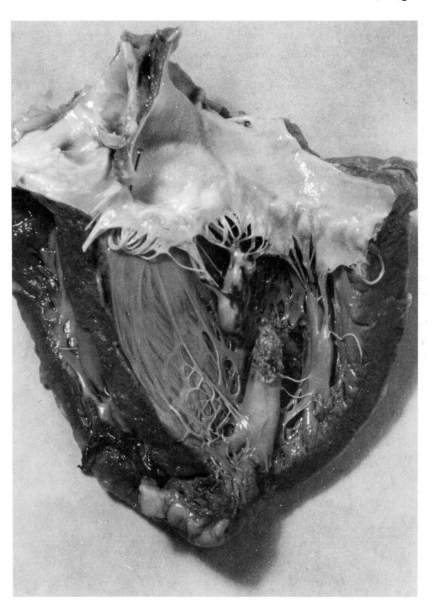

This is the heart of a 64–year–old man who deteriorated rapidly and died, two days after an inferior myocardial infarction.

Q : What is the diagnosis ?

A35.

A :   Ruptured posteromedial papillary muscle

Papillary muscle rupture is an uncommon cause of death following myocardial infarction, accounting for 0.9–5% of all deaths in the immediate post-infarct period. The posteromedial papillary muscle is the more likely muscle to rupture, and is involved in inferior infarcts. The anterolateral muscle is involved in anterolateral infarcts.

This complication may arise even in small infarcts, possibly as a result of potent shear forces operating across a localised area of necrosis.

Presentation is usually early in the course of myocardial infarction and is heralded by cardiovascular collapse, severe pulmonary oedema and signs of torrential mitral regurgitation.

The diagnosis is usually made on transthoracic echocardiography, transoesophageal echocardiography or contrast ventriculography.

The primary differential diagnosis is post-infarct ventricular septal defect. Vasodilatation and intra-aortic balloon pumping may buy time, but definitive treatment must be by surgical repair or mitral valve replacement.

Complete transection of the papillary muscle, as shown in this specimen, is rare. Most papillary muscle rupture involves only one or two heads of an otherwise intact muscle. Complete transection results in rapid haemodynamic deterioration. The pansystolic murmur of mitral regurgitation may not be audible since gross disruption of the mitral valve effectively abolishes any pressure gradient across it. These patients suffer such catastrophic cardiovascular collapse that survival of sufficient duration to reach an operating theatre is virtually unknown.

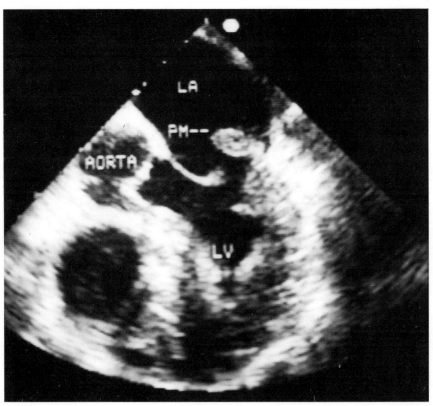

This is the transoesophageal echocardiogram of another patient who sustained a complete transection of a papillary muscle. The flail papillary muscle, in this end-systolic frame, is clearly visible within the left atrial cavity.

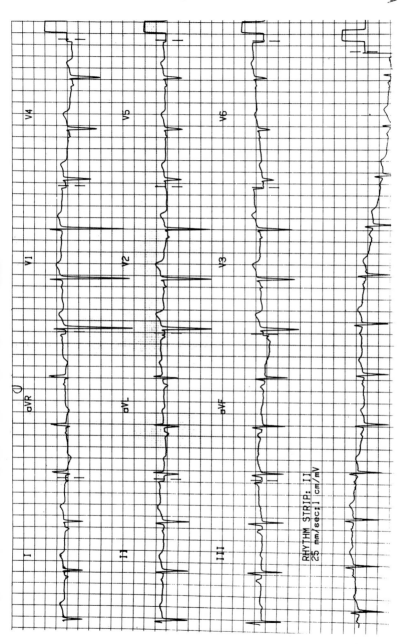

Q: What is the diagnosis ?

A36.

A : Dextrocardia

The mean QRS axis is markedly abnormal. The only positive axial lead is aVR. Some would call this a "north-west" axis, meaning between -90^0 and -180^0. To refer to this as rightward or leftward deviation is largely meaningless.

Why the axis is so abnormal is evident from the precordial leads. The only lead with any significant R wave is V1. Thereafter the precordial leads are strongly negative, and the QRS voltage declines as one progresses across the chest. These abnormalities are highly suggestive of dextrocardia.

Applying the ECG electrodes to the patient in mirror image will yield an entirely normal ECG.

Dextrocardia is a rare abnormality which may be associated with mirror-image transposition of all the viscera (situs inversus totalis). House surgeons should beware the patient with left iliac fossa pain and this ECG – the diagnosis could be appendicitis. More common in the MRCP examination is dextrocardia in the context of Kartagener's syndrome. In this condition there is an abnormality of the dynein arms within cilia, leading to ciliary dysmotility. Patients suffer from chronic sinusitis, bronchiectasis and infertility. The link between ciliary dysmotility and dextrocardia is intriguing but unexplained.

Q37.

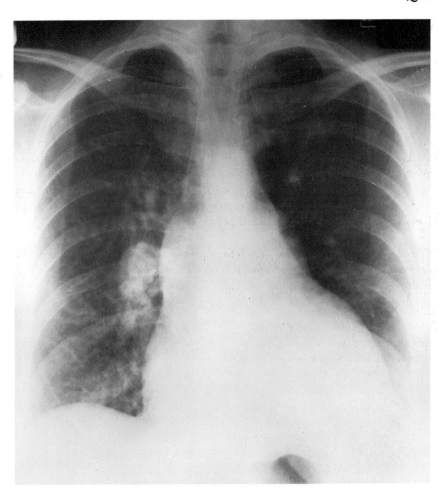

Q :   What does this chest radiograph show ?

A37.

A :   Pulmonary hypertension

On the left heart border, the prominence immediately below the aortic knuckle represents the left pulmonary artery. In this example the left pulmonary arterial shadow is very large and is mirrored by a similar prominence on the right.

The major branches of the main left and right pulmonary arteries are also enlarged. On the right, a compound shadow of the vessels supplying the lower lobe may at first glance be mistaken for a neoplastic lesion. On the left, individual enlarged upper lobe vessels can be seen radiating from the main left pulmonary artery. However, increased vascular markings are not seen at the periphery of the lung fields. This is known as "peripheral pruning" of the pulmonary arterial tree and is characteristic of pulmonary vascular hypertension.

Although these appearances may result from primary pulmonary hypertension, this patient had Eisenmenger's syndrome. It is very unusual for primary lung disease to result in sufficient pulmonary vascular hypertension to give these X-ray appearances.

Q38.

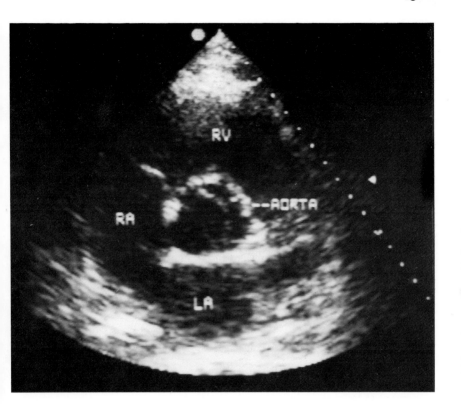

This is a short-axis echocardiographic view at the level of the aortic valve.

Q : What is the abnormality ?

A38.

A :   Bicuspid aortic valve

Instead of the usual tricuspid aortic valve, giving an echo appearance likened to the Mercedes-Benz symbol, this valve has only two cusps.

Bicuspid aortic valves are the commonest congenital cardiac abnormality, affecting about 1% of the population, with a higher incidence in males than females. Although rarely stenotic at birth, bicuspid aortic valves are prone to early calcification during the adult years. This typically results in stenosis of the valve, but can also lead to regurgitation, especially after an episode of infective endocarditis.

The uncomplicated bicuspid aortic valve may produce no abnormal physical findings, or may result in simply an early systolic ejection click, which is easily missed or misinterpreted as a split first sound. In addition, the echocardiographic appearances are often not as convincing as in this example, especially once the valve is calcified and immobile. The diagnosis is therefore most commonly made by the cardiothoracic surgeon, when replacing a stenotic valve in the operating theatre.

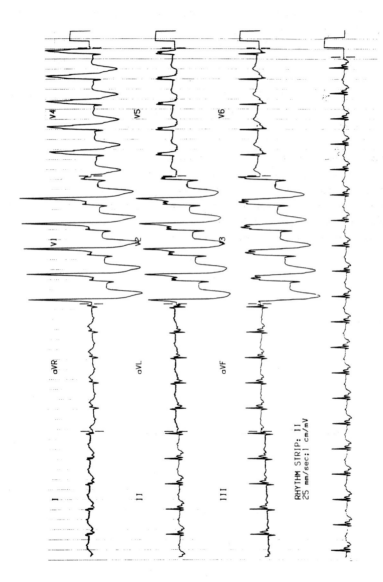

RHYTHM STRIP: II
25 mm/sec; 1 cm/mV

Q: What is the electrocardiographic diagnosis ?

A39.

A :   Right ventricular hypertrophy

Although the QRS complexes are very wide, well in excess of 0.12 seconds, the appearances are far too dramatic to be explained alone by right bundle branch block. The very tall R waves in the early precordial leads, associated with marked abnormalities of repolarisation (ST segment and T wave), are strongly suggestive of right ventricular hypertrophy. Examination of the axial leads reveals borderline right axis deviation. This too is not a feature of lone right bundle branch block.

This patient in fact had Fallot's tetralogy. Note also the long PR interval. The His bundle lies immediately posterior to the membranous VSD of Fallot's and may sometimes be involved.

If the reader has read this book in its logical order it will now be apparent that, apart from right bundle branch block, the more uncommon causes of positive R waves in the early precordial leads are posterior infarction, type A Wolff–Parkinson–White syndrome and right ventricular hypertrophy.

Q40.

The following catheter data are obtained from a cyanosed neonate :

	Pressure (mmHg)	Oxygen saturation (%)
IVC	4	44
RA	3	61
RV	88/1	60
PA	87/62	63
LV	89/0	62
Aorta	86/63	60

Guiding the catheters into place under X-ray screening, the operator was puzzled by some of the catheter positions.

Q : What diagnosis might explain these figures ?

A40.

A :   Transposition of the great arteries

Careful thought is needed to interpret these figures correctly. The pressure data simply show high right-sided pressures, identical to the slightly low left-sided figures. The clue lies in the saturation data. The saturation step-up in the right atrium implies shunting of well-oxygenated blood from the left atrium, through an ASD. However, catheterisation of the left heart fails to detect this well-oxygenated blood.

The explanation is that the left-heart catheter did not in fact enter the left heart at all. The figures obtained from the right- and left-heart catheters are identical because both catheters ended up in the right ventricle. In this condition, the right ventricle gives rise to the aorta, and hence is the ultimate destination for catheters inserted via the venous system or the arterial system.

In the data presented, the "PA" figures were in fact from the aorta, and the "LV" figures from the right ventricle.

Hidden from the probing catheters is the left heart, accepting blood from the pulmonary veins and supplying it to the pulmonary arteries. Needless to say, the blood in this system is very well-oxygenated.

The patient has survived thus far because of mixing of the two circulations at the level of the atria, via an ASD, and also through the ductus arteriosus which may still be patent.

All manner of bizarre plumbing can be seen in the field of congenital heart disease, and the above catheter data could be explained in other ways, for example a double-inlet, double-outlet single ventricle with no pulmonary stenosis, in the presence of partial anomalous pulmonary venous drainage into the right atrium. Transposition of the great arteries is of course more common.

A40.
(cont.)

The management of transposition of the great arteries is necessarily surgical. In "simple" transposition (meaning no ASD or VSD), the connections between the pulmonary and systemic circulations are tenuous, being via a patent ductus arteriosus and a patent foramen ovale. Urgent treatment is needed to preserve life, namely a prostaglandin infusion to maintain patency of the ductus and a balloon atrial septostomy (the Rashkind procedure). This latter procedure involves pulling an inflated balloon through the interatrial septum to create an ASD.

Traditionally, transposition with an ASD (whether congenital or fashioned by balloon septostomy) was treated by a Mustard procedure. In this procedure an intra-atrial "baffle" is positioned, such that saturated blood from the pulmonary veins is channelled into the right atrium (and hence the systemic circulation) while desaturated blood from the venae cavae is channelled the other way. Similarly, transposition with a congenital VSD may be managed with a Rastelli operation, in which the VSD is closed in such a way as to leave the aorta communicating with the left ventricle. The main pulmonary artery is tied off and a conduit from the right ventricle to the pulmonary artery inserted.

The more modern solution to transposition of the great arteries is the arterial switch procedure, in which the great arteries are divided and switched. Though this sounds the ideal solution, the disadvantages are a high early mortality and the need to perform the operation during the first two weeks of life. If the procedure is undertaken after this time, the left ventricle proves incapable of sustaining the systemic circulation.

Q41.

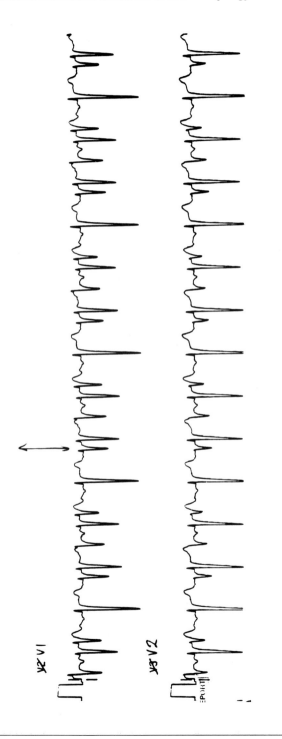

Q :: What is the explanation for this very unusual rhythm strip ?

A41.

A : "Piggy-back" cardiac transplant

Close analysis of this rhythm strip reveals two different morphologies of QRS complex. The spacing between identical complexes is regular but complexes of different morphology bear no temporal relation to one another. Every so often the different complexes are superimposed to form a fusion beat.

This appearance is generated by two separate hearts within the same patient, the result of a "piggy-back" transplant. Instead of the donor organ replacing the recipient's diseased heart, the new heart is added into the circulation to work in tandem with the recipient's. This is an unusual form of cardiac transplant usually performed when the donor organ is too small to supply an adequate cardiac output on its own. The results of this form of transplant are less good than traditional replacement transplantation.